THE WOMAN'S ULTIMATE QUICKSTART GUIDE TO
REVERSING TYPE 2 DIABETES AND TAKING
CHARGE OF YOUR HEALTH

UNVEILING THE TRUTH

SECRETS THEY DON'T WANT
YOU TO KNOW ABOUT
TYPE 2 DIABETES

STEPHANIE GUIGNARD

TABLE OF CONTENTS

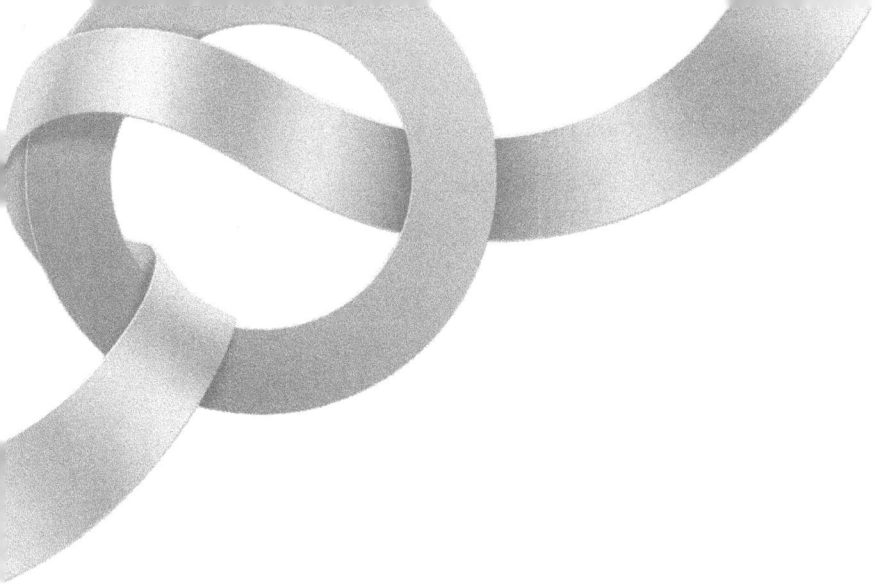

INTRODUCTION

Ever feel like your doctor is treating you like a mystery they don't want to solve? Or that your health is as important to them as finding a needle in a haystack?

Newsflash, my friend, you're not the issue here. You didn't sign up for the Type 2 Diabetes club because you had a childhood love affair with candy or spent too much time playing video games. And nope, it's not because your mom chose the bottle over the breast. You can finally stop blaming yourself for those rebellious teenage years and say sorry to your mom for all the grey hairs. Let's get this straight: **Diabetes is not your fault.**

So, if you've ever been given the cold shoulder by a doctor or made to feel like a dunce for a number on a scale or a blood sugar reading, I'm here to say sorry on their behalf.

In this book, I'll let you in on some juicy insider secrets. Think of it as a behind-the-scenes tour of Diabetes, specially tailored for women. After years of digging deep into research and listening to countless personal stories, I've got some truth bombs to drop.

Buckle up, because it's going to be a wild ride!

Welcome to a special book made just for you. You're here because you or someone close to your heart has something called Type 2 Diabetes. Don't worry, this might sound big and scary, but this book is here to help!

Have you ever felt like there's something more you need to know about Type 2 Diabetes? Like there are secrets that people don't want to share? Well, this book is going to share those secrets with you.

We are going uncover everything "they" don't want us to know. From why your body behaves the way it does, to what foods make you feel good or bad, to how you can still have fun while taking care of yourself!

This book is like a best friend who will hold your hand, and help you understand your body better as it relates to Type 2 Diabetes. Remember, every woman is a queen, and queens are strong. You are stronger than you think and with a little bit of knowledge, you can be in charge of your health.

So, get ready to unlock these secrets and learn how you can feel better and live a happier, healthier life with Type 2 Diabetes. We promise it's going to be a fun journey, full of learning and full of love. So, buckle up, ladies, because knowledge is power and you're about to become very powerful!

Let's get started! Welcome to 'What They Don't Want You To Know About Diabetes.'

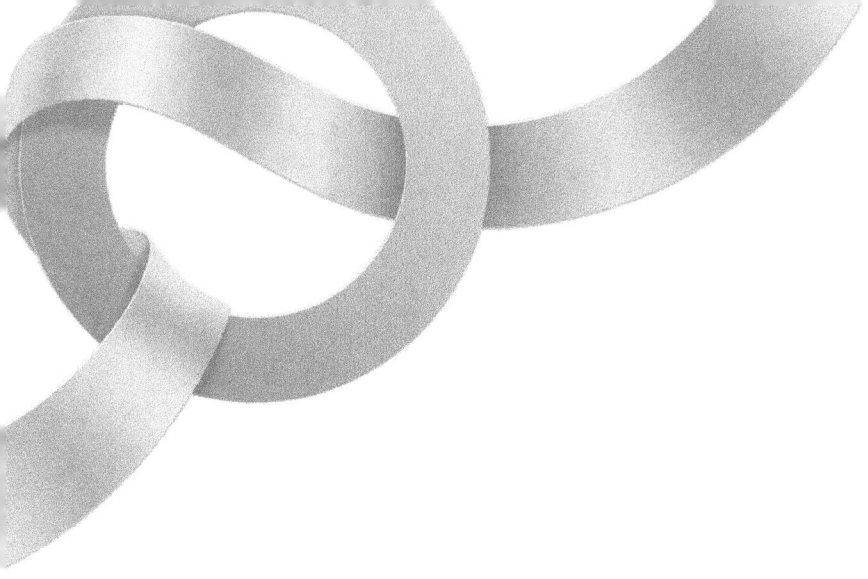

WHAT IS DIABETES?

Imagine your body is like a sugar factory. The machine that controls the sugar is called the pancreas. Now, what happens if there's too much sugar? Our pancreas machine works extra hard, making a helper called insulin to handle it. But sometimes, it gets too tired and can't make enough insulin. That's when the sugar starts to pile up and we call this Type 2 Diabetes. Technical terms, your physician will take some blood during your physical exam and if that number is higher than 126 mg/dl on two separate occasions, a diagnosis of Diabetes will be given. It is a good idea to get blood sugar check when you get your physical exam and every three months get the Hemoglobin A1C checked

You might have heard about Type 1 Diabetes and something called gestational diabetes, but in this book, when we say "Diabetes", we're talking about Type 2 Diabetes.

Now, we're going to learn more about Type 2 Diabetes, like detectives solving a mystery. And you, my Diabetes Maven, are the chief detective!

Our bodies need sugar (also known as glucose) for energy, like cars need fuel to run. We get this sugar from the foods we eat. The helper, insulin, works like a key that opens up our cells to let the sugar in. When we have Type 2 Diabetes, the pancreas machine is too tired to make enough keys. This means the sugar gets stuck outside the cells and starts to build up in our blood.

The building up of sugar is not good for us. It can make us feel tired, thirsty all the time, or make us need to go to the bathroom a lot. Sometimes it might even make our vision blurry. If we don't treat it, it can lead to bigger problems in the long run, like hurting our heart, kidneys, eyes, and nerves.

Remember, having Type 2 Diabetes doesn't mean you've done anything *wrong*. It's something that happens to many people, especially as they get older. Other things that might make it more likely are if it runs in your family, or if you're overweight.

But guess what? There are many things we can do to feel better! Eating healthier foods, moving our body more, and taking medicines if we need them can help manage Type 2 Diabetes. This book will help you understand how to do all these things and more.

So, let's dive deeper into the mystery of Type 2 Diabetes, and discover all the secrets they don't want us to know. Are you ready, chief detective? Let's go!

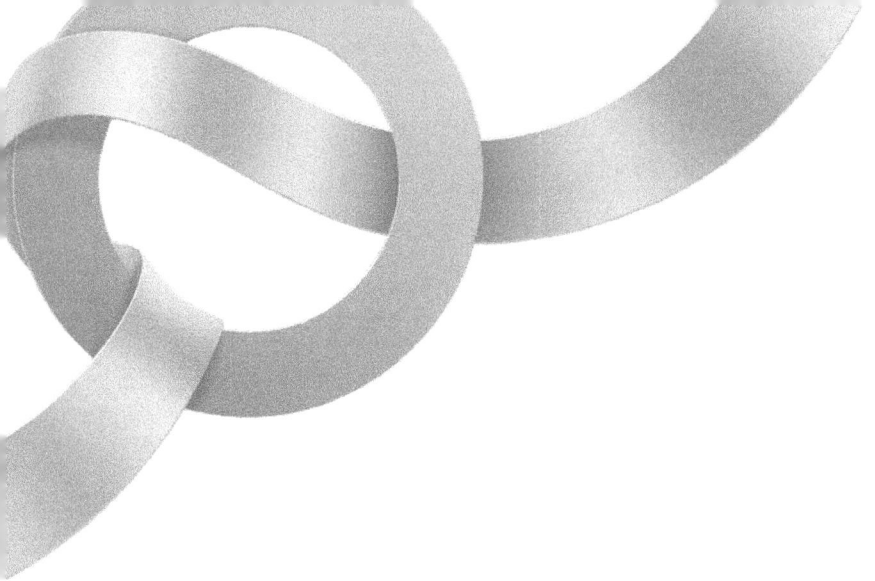

SYMPTOMS OF DIABETES

Let's talk about something that's more elusive than a good mystery novel: the symptoms of diabetes. They're a tricky bunch, often playing hide-and-seek in your body for years without getting caught. So, it's super important to turn into a self-care superstar and get those annual check-ups with your doc.

Think of it as a yearly date with your favorite detective, who's on the case of the sneaky villain, Diabetes. Your doc will run some blood work and if the results are higher than a soap opera star's hairdo a couple of times, you might just have a diabetes diagnosis on your hands.

So, what clues should you be looking out for? Well, it's a laundry list that could fill a soap opera script:

1. A thirst that's more intense than a summer love triangle.

2. Bathroom breaks that are more frequent than commercial breaks during your favorite show.

3. Hunger that rivals your craving for the next episode of your favorite series.

4. Unexpected weight loss that's faster than a reality show transformation.

5. Fatigue that makes you feel like you've binge-watched an entire season overnight.

6. Vision that's blurrier than the plot of a convoluted mystery show.

7. Sores that heal slower than a soap opera character's broken heart.

8. A tingling sensation or numbness in your feet - kind of like that pins-and-needles feeling you get when you're waiting for the season finale.

And if you find yourself feeling light-headed, weak, or nursing a headache after indulging in a feast fit for a TV show Thanksgiving special (think high-carb meals), you may just have another clue that diabetes is trying to sneak onto your set.

Remember, you're the star of your own show, so pay attention to your body and don't let diabetes write the script!

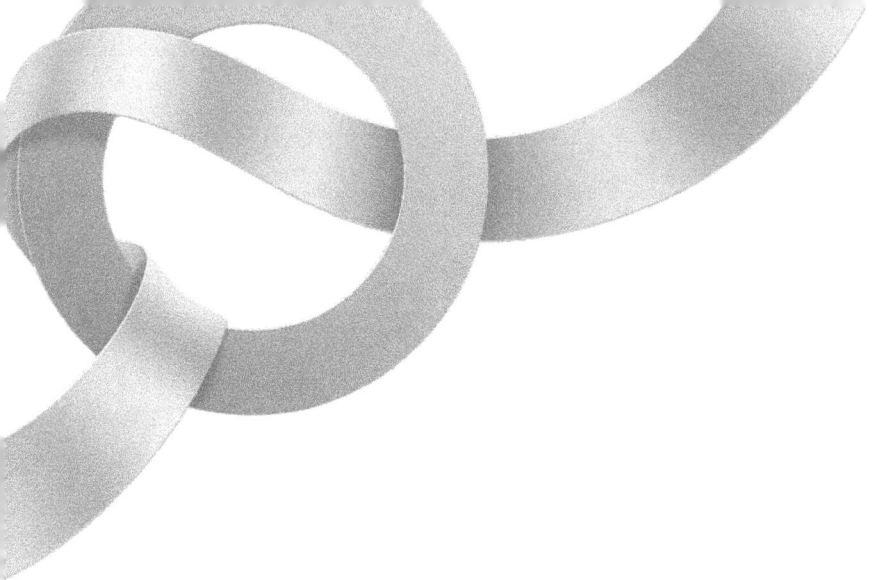

WHAT CAUSES DIABETES?

Ever wondered why some people become the 'chosen ones' for Diabetes, while others remain as untouched as an old VHS tape in a Netflix era? Welcome to the club, friend! It's a mystery that's baffling even the best in the medical biz.

Take Dr. Hyman, for instance. He's got a theory that's more dramatic than a season finale cliffhanger. According to him, the villain is none other than the sweet devil, sugar, and its sinister sidekick, processed food. He says that when you're overweight, you need more sugar to hit that sweet spot of pleasure. And what's the result? You guessed it! You gain more weight, and enter a vicious cycle that's harder to break than a bad TV addiction.

Now, Dr. Hyman believes our insulin receptors (the things that help us process sugar) are as clogged. And the best way to unclog them? Well, he proposes a diet that's as low-carb and vegan as your hipster neighbor's weekend brunch menu.

But wait, there's more! Even though we're as clueless about the exact 'why' of diabetes, there are some factors that make you a hot candidate for the disease.

Topping the list is being overweight or obese, especially if your belly fat is more pronounced. Next comes a sedentary lifestyle – if you're as active as a sloth on a lazy Sunday, you're setting yourself up for risk. Don't forget family history, your race or ethnicity, and age – they all hold a role in this drama, too. Think of them as the supporting cast in the saga of 'Why Did I Get Diabetes?'. So, let's buckle up, embrace the plot twists and stay tuned for more revelations.

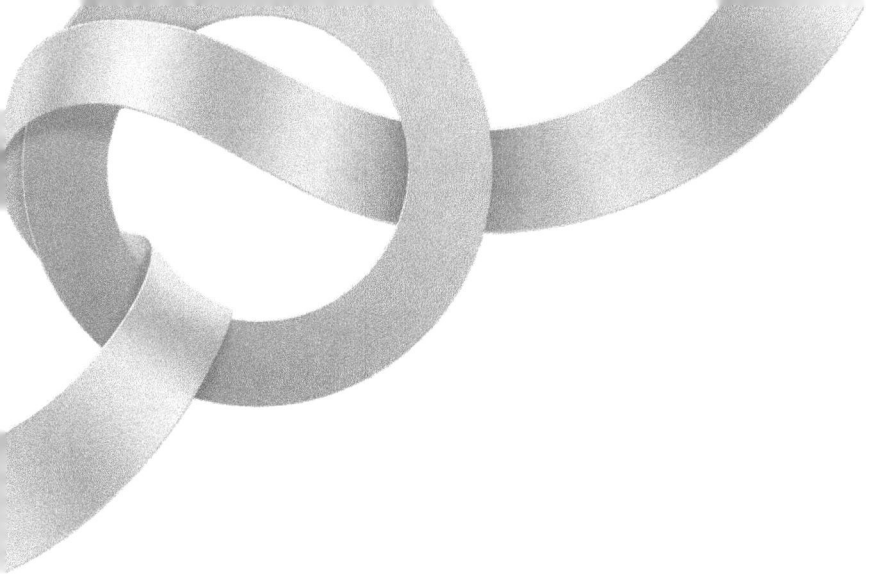

WHAT ARE THE CURRENT TREATMENT OPTIONS FOR DIABETES?

Alright, Mavens, let's talk about some ways we can help our pancreas machine and keep our sugar levels steady.

First up, we have special medicines that we swallow, called antiglycemic medicines. One of the most common ones is called Metformin. These medicines are like helpers that keep our sugar levels from going too high or too low.

Quick heads up, Metformin can dramatically reduce Vitamin D If you are taking Metformin and notice some odd side effects, talk to your doctor.

Next, we have some newer friends in town called GLP-1 medicines. You might hear names like Ozempic and Wegovy. These medicines are like superheroes, they not only help control our sugar levels but also help many people lose weight.

Finally, if our pancreas machine gets too tired and can't make insulin anymore, we might need to take insulin shots. These shots act like the insulin our body used to make, helping sugar get inside our cells.

Remember, every person is different, so what works best for you might not be the same as what works for someone else. Your doctor will help you find the best way to manage your sugar levels.

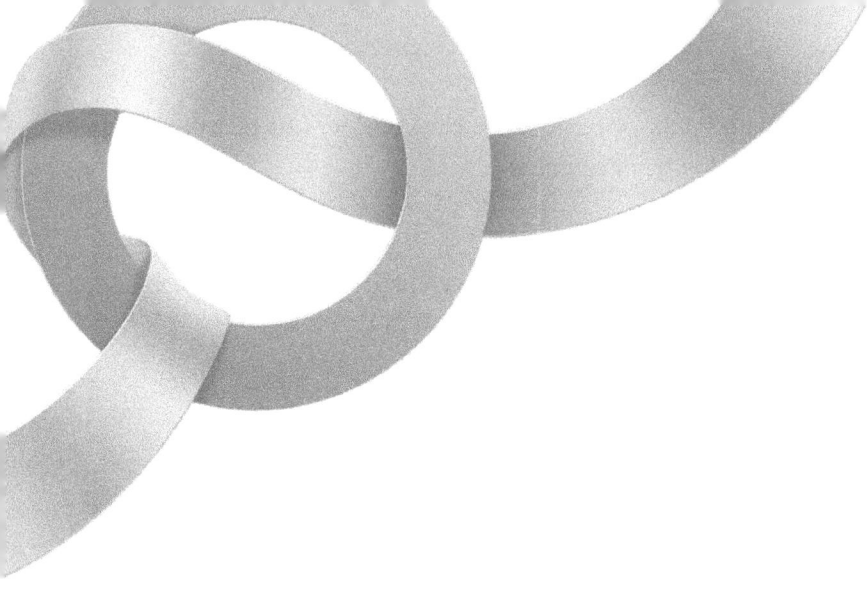

WHAT ARE SOME COMPLICATIONS OF DIABETES?

Did you know that 37 million adults in the U.S., have Type 2 Diabetes? That's as many people as live in a really big city, where I am from, Dallas, TX! But here's a secret clue: 1 in every 5 of these people don't even know they have it. This is because Type 2 Diabetes can be sneaky, like a quiet mouse. You might not feel sick for many years.

Right now, Type 2 Diabetes is like a big, bad villain. It's the 8th biggest cause of people dying in the U.S. And, even though we used to think it was mostly an adult problem, we're now seeing more and more kids being diagnosed because of the big problem we have with obesity.

What makes Diabetes a tricky villain is that it can cause problems in every part of our bodies. It can affect our eyes, making it hard to see. It can hurt our nerves, causing pain or numbness. It can affect our hearts, and even the system that helps us have babies.

But remember, Mavens, every villain can be defeated with the right tools and knowledge. That's what we're going to learn in this book!

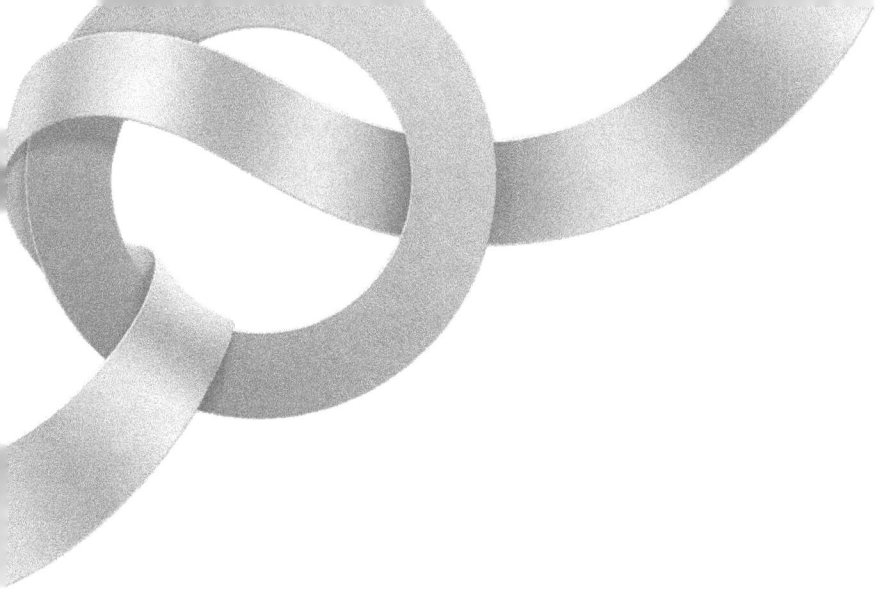

SECRET #1

Through the years, our menu has gone through a radical makeover. Now it's full of chemically enhanced, sugar-stuffed, processed goodies. Think of them as a movie star with too much plastic surgery – they might look good on the outside, but inside? Not so much. The result? Our hormones are throwing a wild party and we're left with the mess.

Meanwhile, we've settled into a comfy, sit-around kind of lifestyle. With the dawn of automobiles and TV dinners, we've all stepped onto the not-so-healthy lane. We're taking in more calories than we're burning, thanks to the sofa's irresistible call. Couch potatoes, unite!

The real culprit here? Our two-faced buddy, sugar. Sugar is like that pesky neighbor who never leaves – it's everywhere, in everything. Even in pickles, for crying out loud! You can't escape it, and the system doesn't want you to.

Every time we munch on something sugary, our poor pancreas is panting in the corner, trying to pump out enough insulin to keep up. It's like running a marathon without any training – a real uphill battle.

Add in some mischievous additives like MSG, extra sodium, and carrageenan, and it's a perfect storm for Diabetes. In a high-stakes game of laboratory Ratatouille, these additives have been caught red-handed causing Diabetes. They're also the sneaky culprits behind weight gain and a higher risk of cancer.

The result? A layer of stubborn belly fat that messes with how our bodies use sugar. It's like having a monkey wrench thrown in your finely tuned machine. And guess who's cheering from the sidelines? Insulin.

Yes, that same insulin we've been talking about is not just snoozing on the job, it's also encouraging fat cells to multiply and stick around, even when we're sweating it out at the gym. It's sending our body the wrong signals, tricking us into thinking we're hungry, while the glucose meant to feed our cells is stuck outside, knocking on the door.

Insulin, you've got some explaining to do!

Remedy:

This stuff is sneakier than a soap opera villain, but we're going to kick it to the curb, one sweet little bite at a time. See, sugar's got this way of getting its hooks in you. It's as addictive as the gossip on daytime TV, making your brain light up like a fireworks display. It's the same kind of buzz folks get from something a lot more sinister - cocaine. So, trying to ditch it cold turkey is like trying to resist a juicy cliffhanger - it's darn near impossible!

But never fear, ladies, I've got a plan for you. Take it slow and steady. Here's the game plan:

1. Get out your detective glasses and start reading labels. Sugar's got more aliases than a fugitive on the run: sucrose, dextrose, glucose, beet sugar, cane sugar, to name a few.

2. Say sayonara to sugary drinks. Opt for water or sparkling water instead. It's like choosing a good book over a bad TV show.

3. Crank up the protein and fat at meal times. They're like the reliable friends who always have your back - they'll keep you full and fend off those sugar cravings.

4. Find your favorite recipes and give them a makeover. Think of it as recasting a role in your favorite show to make it low carb.

5. Become a fruit and veggie fanatic. They're the unsung heroes of your diet, always there to support you.

6. Say no to processed foods and yes to whole foods. It's like choosing real friends over fake ones.

With these tips and tricks up your sleeve, you'll be able to kick sugar to the curb in no time! Now, who's ready to win this fight?

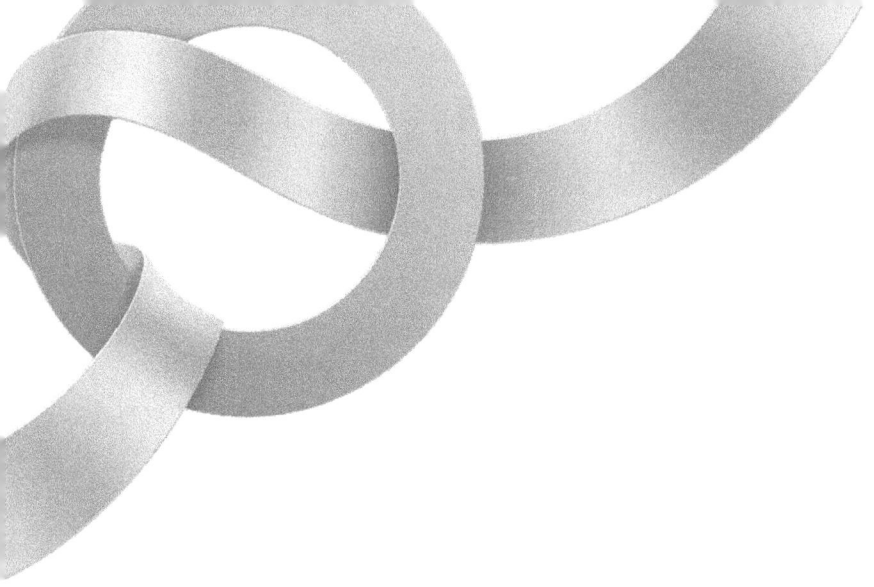

SECRET #2:

Type 2 Diabetes plays favorites. It's like a fashion show where the experience of wearing a dress is totally different from donning pants. For us ladies, it's a whole other ballgame compared to the gents.

Top of the diabetes drama? Heart disease, the biggest, baddest villain of them all. Picture this: Women with diabetes are about four times more likely to tango with heart disease than women without diabetes. For men, they're only twice as likely. Now, that's hardly fair, is it?

But there's more to this twisted tale. If a woman has a heart attack, it's like falling on a patch of ice and not getting up as quickly. All this thanks to a fond farewell to our shield-maiden hormone, estrogen, due to our dear friend, menopause. So, let's tip our hats to menopause for that extra sprinkle of chaos!

You might wonder, why the heart? Well, high blood sugar likes to sneak around, causing mischief and wrecking our precious heart vessels, making the risk of a heart attack skyrocket.

But hold on, the diabetes roller coaster ride doesn't stop there. It throws in a few more gut-wrenching loops for us gals than for guys, like problems with our eyesight, our kidneys, and even bouts of the blues (a.k.a. depression), again thanks to a drop in estrogen. Are you seeing a pattern yet?

What's more, diabetes has a peculiar hit list. Some groups of women get the diabetes 'love' more. This includes our African American, Hispanic, American Indian, Alaska Native, and Asian/Pacific Islander sisters.

Remedy:

Ladies, it's time to guard your hearts and I'm not talking about the defense against the dark arts of bad dates or ghosting exes. No, this is about the ol' ticker, your very own heart.

Exercise. I know, the word alone triggers an allergic reaction in most of us. I mean, who willingly signs up for panting, sweating and feeling like your lungs are staging a revolt? But bear with me, because I have never, in all my life, met a person who finished a workout and said, "Gosh, I wish I hadn't done that."

Sure, I may be the reigning queen of 'Exercise? No thank you!', but even I can't deny the magic of getting moving. So, if you're currently as active as a hibernating bear, don't fret. Start small. A 10-minute post-meal boogie or a brisk walk around the block is all it takes. Remember, if your heart's a-thumpin', you're a-jumpin' in the right direction.

And let's not forget our friends from the garden – fruits and veggies. They come loaded with heart-happy nutrients and make an excellent plus-one to any meal. Consider them your internal suit of armor, defending your heart from the onslaught of unhealthy choices.

Lastly, let's talk stress. It's like that unwelcome house guest who overstays their welcome and eats all your snacks. Show it the door with some daily journaling or meditation. If you can pray away the stress, even better! Not only will this make you feel calmer, but it'll help keep those pesky cortisol levels in check. And a relaxed you equals a happier, healthier heart. Now, isn't that a love story worth striving for?

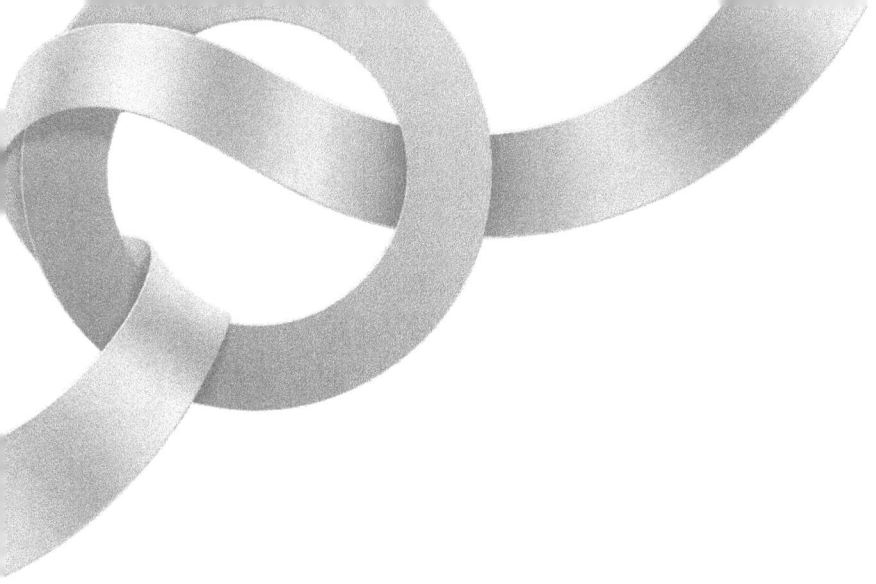

SECRET # 3: SEXUAL HEALING

For women, our bodies go through a cycle every month that can make our blood sugar levels hard to predict. We can have heavier periods and cravings for certain foods that can make it harder to manage our diabetes. As progesterone decreases during a monthly cycle, cravings for carbohydrates increase as this hormone needs glucose to function optimally.

If Blood sugar is too high, it can actually make women have irregular cycles. Having irregular cycles is something you need to talk with your doctor about as too many missed cycles can put you at a higher risk for endometrial cancer.

As if that wasn't enough, Diabetes can also make us less interested in sex or make it less enjoyable. Some women might have dryness down there that can make sex uncomfortable. This can be caused by many things, including nerve damage, less blood flow, medications, and changes in hormones.

After we go through something called menopause, our bodies make less estrogen. This can make our blood sugar levels go up and down unpredictably. We might gain weight, which can mean we need more insulin or other diabetes medicines. Hot flashes and night sweats might interrupt our sleep and make managing blood sugar harder. This is also a time when sex can become more problematic.

Finally, because of higher blood sugar levels, women with diabetes have more yeast infections because yeast feed on high amount of sugar. They love it if this is hanging around in our body. The more the merrier.

Remedy:

Ladies, we're diving into the pot of culinary goodness to talk balanced meals. Now, don't recoil in terror. This isn't an episode of "Attack of the Killer Kale." Instead, it's all about honoring the foodie godmothers of our health, the ever-faithful fruits and veggies.

Think of these colorful morsels as your personal wellness warriors. They're armed with vital nutrients that keep our hormones in line and blood sugar as balanced as a yogi in tree pose. And a bonus, ladies? With sugar levels steadier than a tightrope walker, our monthly cycle runs like clockwork and our internal yeast party goes from raucous rave to mellow book club.

Need a little extra help? Don't shy away from the lube. Like a well-oiled engine, it protects your delicate areas and can elevate 'getting lucky' from a friction burn experience to a slide into home base. It's all about the pleasure, ladies!

And let's not forget about the infamous time of the month when progesterone does a runner, and cravings hit us like a freight train. Plan ahead for these. Stock your pantry with protein and fats so you're prepared for the sugar-seeking missiles your body launches. Remember, the more prepared you are, the less likely you are to dive headfirst into a tub of ice cream at 3 AM.

So, there you have it, folks. The route to a healthier, happier you is through your stomach. Now, who's ready for a salad?

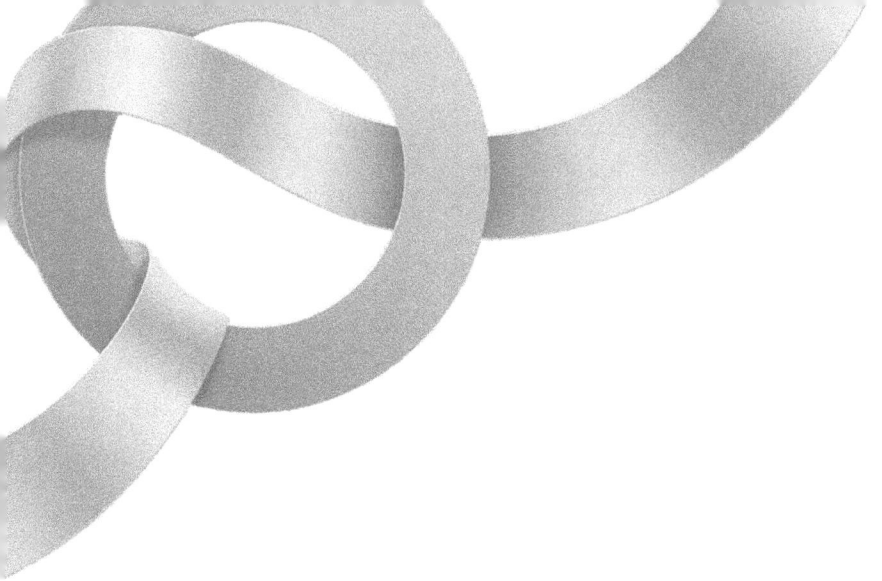

SECRET # 4: STRESSED OUT

Alright, buckle up, because we're about to dive into the thrilling world of another hormone that just loves to stir the pot. Meet Cortisol, the unpredictable wild child of our hormonal family.

Cortisol is our body's action hero, leaping into action when danger looms. Picture this: you're strolling through the woods, humming a tune, when out pops a bear. Your cortisol levels zoom up like a roller coaster hitting its peak. Its job? To help your body hightail it out of there. The catch? This adrenaline-fueled escapade triggers a spike in blood sugar to fuel the grand escape. Talk about a plot twist!

But wait, there's more. Cortisol isn't just about daring escapes. It's also the puppet master of our metabolism and blood pressure. In short bursts, it's like a health-boosting elixir, powering up our immune system by putting a leash on inflammation. But let it hang around too long, and the party crashes. Prolonged cortisol presence turns into inflammation and a slump in our immune system. Oh, the irony!

Now let's talk about our sleep. See, cortisol loves a good routine. It normally chills out as we tuck in for the night, then revs up in the morning to get us up and running. But toss in some sleep loss or a wonky sleep pattern, and cortisol goes off the rails, throwing a wrench in the works.

The moral of the story? Cortisol is like that rich dessert we all love – a little is divine, but too much and we're groaning with regret. Balance is key, so let's not overindulge, shall we?

Remedy:

Alright ladies, it's time to take a deep breath, unwind, and show that bossy cortisol who's really in charge! Now, don't start stress-sweating at the thought of it - I promise it's easier than assembling IKEA furniture.

The game plan? Well, it's all about relaxation techniques. Picture this: you're a mindfulness ninja, armed with deep breaths and meditation, ready to kick that cortisol to the curb. Start your day with a prayer - or meditation if that's your jam. You could even do interpretive dance if that floats your boat. The key here is to get into a Zen state that would make a Buddhist monk proud.

Now, to round off your day, it's all about journaling. Scribble down everything that brought you joy. Maybe it was your dog's silly antics, or the free coffee from the café, or finally managing to keep a houseplant alive (congrats!). Studies show that when we focus on our joy, we release those happy hormones, like your brain's own brand of mood-boosting confetti, leaving cortisol sobbing in a corner.

In essence, it's all about turning stress-busting into a daily habit. Consider it a workout for your mental health. But unlike that forgotten gym membership, this is one routine you won't want to skip. So go ahead, deflate that cortisol balloon, and feel the peace (and hilarity) descend.

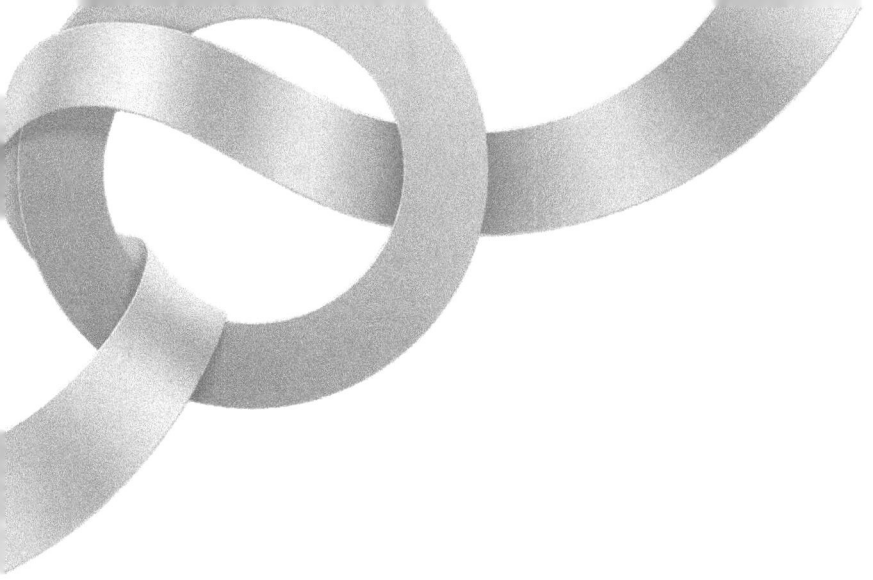

SECRET #5: PUT IT IN REVERSE

Brace yourselves, ladies, because the final secret is set to make your jaws drop! So far, it's felt like we're stuck in a gloomy weather forecast, hasn't it? But wait! There's a silver lining to this diabetes cloud. This isn't a soap opera, and diabetes doesn't have to hog the spotlight. We can demote it to a cameo and live our lives in the freedom we deserve.

Here's the shocker that the white coats might not have shared: Diabetes can be reversed! Gasp! I know, it's like finding out your favorite soap star isn't leaving the show. I remember when I got the diagnosis. I figured it was curtains for me. Either a heart attack or cancer would be my final act. Then, I spotted the light at the end of the tunnel. One game-changer turned it all around, and I believe it can do the same for you. Yes, Diabetes is a bit like a theatre troupe affecting the whole body. Changing that requires a whole stage full of adjustments. But remember, Rome wasn't built in a day. One step at a time is the way to go. For me, it all started with meal times.

Believe it or not, intermittent fasting helped me shed the pounds, stabilized my blood sugar, and brought my A1C levels back on track. And no, I didn't have to bid farewell to my beloved foods. It was all about timing. Our bodies don't need a midnight feast, folks. Late-night snacking can lead to weight gain, and the later you eat, the more insulin joins the party. So, I started timing my carb-heavy meals around lunch or at least a few hours before bedtime. This simple change was a total game-changer for me.

This is just one of many tips and tricks that worked for me and tons of other folks. So, if your doctor ever tells you that you can't kick Diabetes to the curb, remember my words. You can reverse it with a few changes, a dash of patience, and a sprinkling of perseverance. Will it be a walk in the park? No! Is it worth it? Absolutely! You, my friend, are worth it.

Here's hoping this book has turned on the lightbulb for you and demystified some of the strange things you might have been experiencing. My dream is to arm every woman with the weapons they need to defeat Diabetes once and for all.

And if you'd like to join forces, come on over to our community of thriving women just like you. We're all in this together, after all.

www.ingramcontent.com/pod-product-compliance
Lightning Source LLC
Chambersburg PA
CBHW072224290526

45794CB00007B/2877